Y0-BQB-843

Making Hay

Kenneth Jernigan
Editor

A KERNEL BOOK

published by
NATIONAL FEDERATION OF THE BLIND

ISBN 0-9624122-5-2

Printed in the United States of
America

TABLE OF CONTENTS

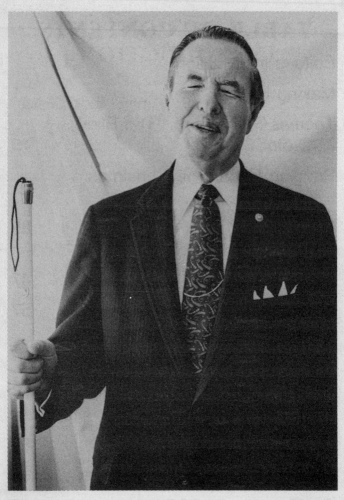

Kenneth Jernigan, President Emeritus
National Federation of the Blind

EDITOR'S INTRODUCTION

This is the fourth Kernel Book. When we started the series a little over two years ago, we didn't know where it would go or how it would be received. The response has exceeded all expectations.

As readers of the series know, I have been the spokesman for the National Federation of the Blind for more than twenty years. Before 1991 total strangers were always stopping me on the street or in the supermarket or airport to ask me what blindness was like. They would tell me that they had seen me on television. They still do it—but more often than not, they now couple their questions with comments about what they have read in one or another of the Kernel Books. They not only talk about things I have told them about my own experiences (both as child and adult) but also about the experiences and lives of others they have met through these pages. They feel that they know us personally and that because of this personal acquaintance they have gained new understanding about blindness.

This, of course, is what I hoped would happen, and it is what I hope will continue to happen as you read the present volume. You will meet new people in this fourth Kernel Book, and you will renew old acquaintances. I have also taken the opportunity (editors are like that) to tell you some additional things about myself—how I tried to break away from the confinement of an isolated existence on a Tennessee farm and what I did as a blind child to try to earn my own way.

As in former volumes, those who appear in this book are people that I know—former students, colleagues in the National Federation of the Blind, and personal friends. There is one exception. I did not know the blind senator Thomas Gore. However, since his great-grandson has now been elected Vice President of the United States, it seems particularly appropriate to include his story. Beyond that, after I graduated from high school and was entering manhood in Tennessee, I used to hear the Vice President's father (Congressman Albert Gore, the Congressman from my district) speak on the radio every Sunday morning. I felt that I knew him personally, and I also feel a personal acquaintance and kinship with his ancestor, who (at least, so far as I know) was the first blind member of Congress.

As to the future of the Kernel Book series, there seems little doubt that we will continue it. The fact that it has already run to a publication of more than two million copies underscores the interest and demand. Meanwhile I hope you will enjoy the present volume and that you will find it interesting and useful.

The essence of its message is simple: We who are blind are pretty much like you. We are, that is, if we have the chance to try. We have our share of both geniuses and jerks, but most of us are somewhere between—ordinary people living regular lives.

Kenneth Jernigan
Baltimore, Maryland
1993

WHY LARGE TYPE

The type size used in this book is 14 Point for two important reasons: One, because typesetting of 14 Point or larger complies with federal standards for the printing of materials for visually impaired readers, and we wanted to show you exactly what type size is necessary for people with limited sight.

The second reason is because many of our friends and supporters have asked us to print our paperback books in 14 Point type so they too can easily read them. Many people with limited sight do not use Braille. We hope that by printing this book in a larger type than customary, many more people will be able to benefit from it.

MAKING HAY

by Kenneth Jernigan

As a blind child growing up on a farm in the hills of Middle Tennessee in the late 1920's and early 1930's, I did a lot of thinking. This is not surprising since there wasn't much else to do. We lived in a four-room house on a gravel road, and I doubt that an automobile a week passed our door. We had no radio, no telephone, no newspaper, no magazines, and no books except the Bible and the textbooks my brother (four years older than I) brought home from school.

The world of the late '20's and early '30's in rural Tennessee was a totally different place from what we know today. Nobody thought about atom bombs, pollution, or jet planes. About the hottest topic I heard discussed by my elders was whether it was a sin for a woman to bob her hair and what the likelihood was that you would go to hell if you played cards. I had better explain that last remark. I am not referring to playing cards for money, just ordinary games around the family table. And while we are on the subject, there was no question at all about whether you would go to hell if you danced or played pool. You would.

The difference between the world of then and there and the one of here and now was not limited to the rural areas. Let me give you an example. When I went off to the Tennessee School for the Blind in Nashville at the age of six (that would have been January of 1933), one of the more charming customs of the place was a Saturday morning ritual involving the Scriptures. Shortly after breakfast the small boys (I don't know what happened to the girls since there was strict segregation) were plopped down on a bench and given the task of memorizing a chapter from the Bible. It didn't do any good to protest, object, or try to resist. You sat there until you memorized it, after which you were free to go play.

One's religion had nothing to do with it, nor did one's interest or aptitude. When you got the task done, you could (within limits) go where you pleased and do what you liked. Meanwhile you couldn't. And whatever time you spent trying to beat the system was just that much of the morning gone. I suppose I need not tell you that I quickly concluded to learn my chapter with minimum delay, which I religiously (no play on words intended) did. As a result, I have been a devout Bible quoter ever since—and much, I might add, to my benefit and long-range satisfaction. Ah, well, children are not always in the best position to know what will stand them in good stead.

I don't want to leave you with the impression that everything in that Tennessee world of the '20's and '30's concerned the Bible or religious matters. It didn't. We popped corn in a pan of bacon grease on the wood stove in the kitchen or in a long-handled popper at the fireplace in one or the other of the two bedrooms. (The house had a kitchen, a dining room, and two bedrooms.) We visited our neighbors and relatives, either walking or (if the distance was too far) riding in a wagon drawn by two mules; we gathered hickory nuts and walnuts; and now and again the family sang songs or listened to a neighbor play a banjo. At Christmas time there was a great deal of cooking, but no convenience foods, of course, and as little as possible bought from the store. For instance, we didn't make fruit-cake. That would have cost too much. Instead, we made jam cake. The black walnuts, the homemade blackberry jam, and most of the other ingredients came from our farm and required no outlay of cash.

As to my personal situation, it was (if you want to be high-toned about it) what you might call anomalous. Nobody in the neighborhood had ever known a blind person, so there was no one to give advice. My parents loved me, but they didn't know what to do. This led to some strange inconsistencies. For instance, my mother and dad didn't want me to carry wood for the fireplace or stove or water from the spring, which was only a few feet from the house. They didn't want me to play in the yard or go any farther than the porch. They were afraid I might get hurt. Yet, they had no objection at all to my shooting firecrackers at Christmas time.

It was regarded as a natural thing for boys in that part of the country to shoot firecrackers, and I suppose my parents just never thought about it. One of my earliest memories is of me standing on the front porch with a match and a firecracker in my hand and of my father, saying as he went past me into the house, "You'd better be careful, or you'll blow your hand off with that thing." Young as I was, I knew that he was right and that nobody would stop me if I was careless—so I wasn't careless. I developed a technique of holding the match just below the head and pressing the firecracker fuse against it. Match and fuse were held between my thumb and index finger, so there was no possibility of the firecracker's exploding in my hand since my fingers were between it and the flame. Never once did I get hurt, and I think the experience helped me learn something about risk taking and proper caution.

As I have already said, I did a lot of thinking as I was growing up. I also did a lot of planning, for I didn't want to spend the rest of my life in close confinement in that four-room house on the farm. As I reasoned it, I needed to read all the books I could, and I needed to go to college. Therefore, as Braille and recorded books became available to me through the books for the blind program of the Library of Congress, I followed through on the matter and crammed my head as full of book learning as I could. Later I went to college and put the limited environment of the farm behind me.

Meanwhile, I wanted to do productive work and make some money. This wasn't easy since my family (though loving me) thought I was virtually helpless. My first effort (caning chairs at the School for the Blind) brought more labor than cash, but I had to start where I could. Also, we had cows on the farm, and we sold their milk to a nearby cheese factory. During summer vacations I milked cows night and morning and got ten cents a week for it. At the time I was probably eleven or twelve.

During the first part of the Second World War (I would have been fourteen or fifteen), I made a little money collecting peach seeds. I sold them to a man who came by twice a week in a truck. I was told that the kernels were used for filters in gas masks, but I don't know whether that was true or not. What I do know is that I got a penny a pound for them and that there were a tremendous number of peaches eaten in the neighborhood.

Then, there was the NYA (the National Youth Administration), one of Franklin Roosevelt's New Deal programs. Beginning in 1943 I washed windows, scrubbed floors, shined the small boys' shoes, and did other chores at the School for the Blind for three dollars a month—fifteen hours at twenty cents an hour. I thought I was rich.

And there was even an extra dividend. I was not the only boy at the School for the Blind who got three dollars a month for working for the NYA. There were quite a number, which meant that we now had a cash economy, with more money in circulation than the boys at the School for the Blind had ever known. It stimulated business. I was one of those who profited. I established a relationship with a local wholesale house and walked there once or twice a week to carry large boxes of candy and chewing gum back to the School. I bought the candy for three cents a bar and sold it for a nickel. Going for the candy was not only good exercise but also good profit. My roommate and I did a thriving business. It helped me get some of the money to start to college.

There was also my broom-making project. A neighbor in the country raised broom corn, and I took it with me to the School for the Blind and made it into brooms. (All blind boys in those days were taught chair caning and broom making regardless of their aptitudes or wishes, and I think I could still do a creditable job at either task.) My neighbor supplied the broom corn, and I made and sold the brooms. We split the profits.

During the latter part of the Second World War (by this time I was sixteen or seventeen) I got a chance during the school year to make some money by sorting aircraft rivets. The Vultee Aircraft Company established a plant near Nashville to make dive bombers, and there were many thousands of rivets in each plane. The workers would drop rivets on the floor; and when the dirt, cigarette stubs, and other leavings were swept up, the assorted mixture was brought to the students at the School for the Blind for sorting. We separated the rivets from the trash, sorted them into sizes and types, discarded any with rough spots on them, and sent them back to the aircraft plant. It was a messy job, but it was a way to make some money. I think I got two and a half cents a pound for it.

But all of these various jobs were preliminary to my first truly big opportunity. It happened like this: In the summer of 1944 (I was seventeen) I wanted to expand my horizons. Farm laborers in our neighborhood made $1.25 per day, working from sunrise to sunset, and I wanted to join their ranks. The pivotal event occurred when they began making hay. We had no power machinery. There was a mule-drawn mower, and after the hay was cut, there was a mule-drawn rake. The men would follow the rake with pitchforks, putting the hay into shocks and then tossing it into the mule-drawn wagon. Then it would be taken to the barn and put into the loft.

I tried to get my dad and the other decision makers to let me try my hand at making hay. They were not only unwilling but didn't even want to talk about it. In fact when I insisted, they indicated to me that they were busy and had work to do and that I should stop bothering them.

Since I was unwilling to spend the summer doing nothing, I looked around for other opportunities. It occurred to me that I might try my hand at making furniture. Lumber was cheap in those days, and I also had the idea of using spools. At that time thread was wound on wooden spools, plastic not yet having come into use, and almost everybody sewed. Spools were throw-aways, and I got all my relatives, plus department stores in surrounding towns, to save them for me. I got them in every conceivable size and then sorted them and strung them on iron rods to make table legs.

The design was simple, but the product was both durable and graceful. I could make a table in a day and could sell it for $10. It cost me $1.75 in materials, so I had a profit of $8.25. My rejection became a triumph. While the men did back-breaking labor in the hay fields for $1.25 a day, I stayed in my workshop, listened to recorded books, and produced tables for a profit of $8.25. No matter how fast I made them, I could never keep up with demand. It was as regular as clock work—$8.25 net profit day after day, not the $1.25 I would have made in the hay field.

I also designed and made floor lamps from spools. The lamp had an old steering wheel for a base with a pipe running up the center, surrounded by four columns of spools, with a fixture and shade on top. I

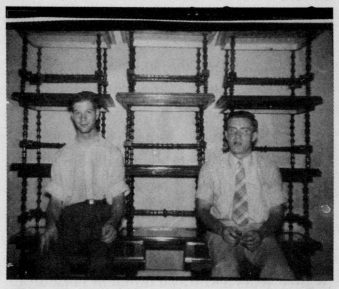

Kenneth Jernigan and a friend in 1945 with tables he designed and built.

could make it in a day, and I sold it for $25, with a cost for materials of a little over $8. This was twice as much profit as I made from a table. The trouble was that the lamps were harder to sell, so I got relatively few orders.

By the end of the summer I had more money than I had ever seen, and I did it again the following year. I went to college in 1945 and never returned to the furniture business, but it taught me a valuable lesson, as did the other jobs I have described. There are many ways to make hay, and if you lose $1.25, you may make $8.25 if you put your mind to it. As I have already said, the world of fifty years ago was a different place from the world of today—but many of the lessons still hold. They probably always will, and one of them is that making hay is a lifelong process.

THOMAS PRYOR GORE: "THE BLIND ORATOR"

by Sharon Gold

*In 1976 the National Federation of the Blind's magazine, the **Braille Monitor,** published a series of profiles of distinguished blind Americans in celebration of the nation's bicentennial. One of these profiles was of Thomas Pryor Gore, the first blind United States Senator. Sharon Gold, President of the National Federation of the Blind of California, did the research and wrote the profile. Since Senator Gore was the great-grandfather of our newly-elected Vice President, it seems fitting to include it in this Kernel Book. Here it is:*

Thomas Pryor Gore, the first totally blind man to sit in the United States Senate, was born on December 10, 1870, in Old Choctaw (later known as Webster) County,

Mississippi. His father, Thomas Madison Gore, who served as a soldier in the Confederate Army during the Civil War, was a farmer and a lawyer.

An accident at the age of eight resulted in the total loss of sight in one of Gore's eyes and severe injury to the other eye, causing him to be totally blind at the age of eleven. Gore continued his studies in the public schools of Walthall, Mississippi, his classmates and members of his family reading his lessons aloud to him. After graduating from high school in 1888, he studied two additional years, taking a scientific course.

In 1890 Gore graduated from a normal school [a two-year teacher-training institution], obtained a teaching license, and taught in a public school during the year 1890-1891. He then entered Cumberland University in Lebanon, Tennessee, as a student in the School of Law. Shortly after Gore's graduation with an LL.B. degree in 1892, he was admitted to the bar and began practicing law in Walthall. As a boy Gore had spent a year serving as a page in the Mississippi Legislature, and throughout his school years he had read and studied political economy, the writings of Thomas Jefferson, and any works he could procure on the art and science of government. In 1891 he was nominated for the State Legislature but was forced to withdraw his nomination because he was under age.

Gore, like his father and other relatives, became an active member of the Populist Party and was soon considered the best-known and most able stump speaker for that party. When the Mississippi Populists were defeated in 1895, the "Blind Orator," as he had come to be known, moved to Corsicana, Texas, where he continued to be an active member of the Populist Party and practiced law.

In 1896 he served as a delegate to the Populist National Convention in Saint

Louis, Missouri, and two years later was defeated as a candidate for the U.S. Congress on the People's Party Ticket. After this Gore devoted much of his time to national politics and became affiliated with the Democratic Party in 1899. In 1901, following his new allegiance to the Democratic Party, Gore and his wife, Nina Kay, the daughter of a Texas cotton planter, whom he married on December 27, 1900, joined those pioneers who were moving northward to the new Territory of Oklahoma. They settled in Lawton, where Gore opened a law practice and made his permanent home.

Gore's driving ambition, his superb oratorical ability, and the support of the powerful *Daily Oklahoman* in Oklahoma City, soon made the "Blind Orator" a leading politician in the Oklahoma Territory. In 1902, just one year after settling in the Territory, Gore was elected to the Territory Council and served as a member from 1903 to 1905. In 1907, when the Oklahoma and

Indian Territories joined to form the new State of Oklahoma, Gore assisted with the writing of the State Constitution and was elected one of its first Senators.

He was reelected for two more terms, serving until 1921. During these terms of service in the United States Senate, Gore was especially interested in legislation affecting the farmer and the Indian and was credited with having saved $30 million in royalties for the Indians by filibustering against a resolution giving private individuals oil lease rights.

During the pre-World War I period Gore was one of the progressive members of the Senate, opposing the trusts, high United States tariff rates, and monopolies, especially the railroads. An important and longtime supporter of Woodrow Wilson as a Presidential candidate, Gore helped get Wilson elected in 1912 and endorsed his domestic legislative program. However, with the coming of World War I, Gore decided to oppose

Wilson's foreign policy and America's eventual entry into the war in 1917.

During the war Gore argued against military conscription and pensions, the food administration, emergency governmental control of transportation and communication facilities, and deficit financing. His opposition to Wilson's wartime policies and this country's entry into the League of Nations brought about Gore's defeat by a Wilson supporter in the Democratic primary of 1920.

Gore knew that many of his convictions were unpopular with a large number of his constituents, but being a statesman in preference to a politician, he refused to alter his positions. Thus he returned to private law practice in 1921. In 1930 Gore was again nominated for Senator from Oklahoma and returned to the Senate for a final term from 1931 to 1937.

During this period Gore rose in opposition to policies of both a Republican and a

Democratic President. He was a strong opponent of Franklin D. Roosevelt's social measures, which Gore considered would lead to an over-centralization of government, thus interfering with individual initiative and enterprise. He was opposed to deficit spending.

For a second time in his career as a Senator, his opposition to the policies of a popular President was responsible for his defeat during his 1936 bid for re-election. He spent the final thirteen years of his life practicing law in Washington, D.C., where he specialized in taxes and Indian affairs.

Throughout his political and professional life, Thomas P. Gore was a noted debater and public speaker. His Senate speeches were well-prepared and carefully documented. In preparation for a speech his wife or friends would read to him from books and articles pertaining to the subject on which he was to speak, from his own library of fifty thousand books or at the Library of

Congress. He would then prepare his speech in private.

In addition to his other credits, Gore attended the Democratic National Conventions of 1908, 1912, 1928, and 1936 as a delegate-at-large. He traveled widely throughout the United States, sometimes alone, and always carried one or two books with him which he would ask to have read to him after he became acquainted with people. He died on March 16, 1949, in his Washington apartment, three weeks after suffering a cerebral hemorrhage. He is buried in Oklahoma City's Rose Hill Cemetery.

Thomas Pryor Gore had two children: a daughter, Nina, the mother of the prominent American author, Gore Vidal; and a son, Thomas Notley Gore, father of Albert Gore, U.S. Senator from Tennessee, 1952-1970 [and grandfather of Vice President Gore].

BRINGING HOME THE CHRISTMAS TREE

by Marc Maurer

Marc Maurer is a husband and a father. He is an attorney. He is also blind. He is a man of determination, sensitivity, integrity, and hope. I am glad he is all of these things, for he is also President of the National Federation of the Blind. To a great extent the well-being of future generations of blind people depends upon the National Federation of the Blind and the personal qualities of its leadership. With Marc Maurer leading the organization I am content to have it so. Read "Bringing Home the Christmas Tree," and I think you'll agree with me.

Christmas was for me the most wonderful holiday of the year when I was a boy. There were many small surprises and much happiness.

Thanksgiving was memorable because I was able to come home from the school for the blind which I attended for the first five years of grade school to be with my family. There was always an enormous basket of fresh fruit as well as a huge bowl of nuts to be cracked and eaten. But the best part about Thanksgiving was that it signified the beginning of the Christmas season. Before Thanksgiving, it was simply autumn. After Thanksgiving, Christmas was on its way.

My Christmas problem was to find a way to obtain suitable gifts for my family and friends. My allowance—the weekly grant from my father—just was not large enough to meet all of the demands. When I was small, it was a nickel. By the time I had reached high school, it had grown to the grand sum of a dollar.

When I was in the ninth grade (or maybe it was the tenth), I persuaded the newspaper to put me on as the only blind paper boy in town. Every morning—all three hundred sixty-five days of the year—I rose at five o'clock to collect my papers, deliver them, and walk home. The distance covered in the round trip was a little over two miles.

I liked the walk—especially in the midst of a snow storm. When the wind was blowing, and the snow was falling, I felt humble. It seemed to me that God was reminding us that He had created the world and everything in it.

The paper route brought in a little extra money—as I remember it, between four and five dollars a week. The increase in my financial well-being seemed dramatic.

During the summers I could mow lawns or do other odd jobs. One time I was hired at a dollar an hour to roof a garage. The work was completed in twenty-nine hours. But these summertime activities didn't help at Christmas.

It was all right to begin thinking about Christmas the day after Thanksgiving. However, planning for the most important holiday of the year before the season arrived was out of the question. In my home town Christmas decorations were hung in the streets before Thanksgiving, but our family ignored them until the proper time.

The Christmas season was special and had to be saved until using it was appropriate. This meant that I could not purchase Christmas presents before Thanksgiving. Therefore, I had available only those resources which could be mustered between Thanksgiving and Christmas. Sometimes the money ran out. Nevertheless, gifts must be procured. But, buying them was not essential. They could be manufactured, and sometimes they were.

One year I fashioned a wooden rifle for one of my brothers. Another time I baked homemade Christmas rolls for a friend around the corner. Bread making was a skill I acquired early. And I was not the only one in my family who turned lovingly to handicrafts for the Christmas season. One of my most treasured Christmas presents was a hand-made wooden desk designed and built by my father. I used it for almost ten years.

Part of the delight of the Christmas season was that many unusual things occurred. Visiting neighbors, friends, and relatives came unexpectedly; mysterious packages arrived with contents that must remain secret until the great day; plates of goodies were presented that had been made in a kitchen whose customs were not the same as our own. The cookies and cakes were not the same as the familiar standbys I had come to know so well, and some of them were extraordinarily good.

I was the second of six children and the only member of the family who was blind. My sister and my four brothers attended school in our home town. From the time I was six years old until I was eleven, I attended the school for the blind. At Christmas for two weeks—or a little more—we who were students would say goodbye to the routine at this residential school.

At the school for the blind the wake-up bell rang at 6:30 in the morning. By 6:55 we were expected to be dressed with our faces washed and our teeth brushed. At that time, we lined up to march from the dormitory to the dining hall for breakfast. Breakfast began at 7:00 and lasted half an hour. Between 7:30 and 8:00, we were expected to clean our rooms and make our beds. My roommate and I divided up the cleaning chores. I dusted the furniture while he dusted the floor. Classes began at 8:00 and continued until noon. We marched in line to lunch, which also lasted half an hour.

After lunch we were free to play on the playground for a few minutes. Classes in the afternoon started at 1:00 and finished at 4:00. One period each day was devoted to gym class. After the 4:00 o'clock adjournment of classes we were free to play until we marched to the dining hall at 5:25. After supper there was an hour of mandatory study hall. Then for an hour we could read or play or do as we pleased. By 8:30 all students were supposed to be in their rooms, and at 8:45 the bell rang for lights out.

Two nights a week at the school for the blind there were special events. On Wednesdays and Saturdays we were expected to bathe, and (before bath time) we were permitted to go to the basement of the dormitory for "snack bar." Snack bar was the name for the student-run store. At the snack bar we could buy candy bars, ice cream bars, and a limited selection of penny candy. A prepackaged ice cream cone that had been dipped in chocolate and nuts (we called it a drumstick) cost fifteen cents. I didn't have fifteen cents very often, so my visits to the snack bar were infrequent.

On Saturday the schedule for meals was the same as it was for the rest of the week, but after our rooms had been cleaned and our shoes were polished, the remainder of the day was free. On Sunday we were expected to dress in our Sunday clothes, and we were then sent to church.

When the Christmas holidays came, all of this changed. At home there was no scheduled time to wake up, no pre-set moment for breakfast, no routine for dusting the furniture and making the bed. Furthermore, there were family members to play with, and there were the exciting and mysterious Christmas activities. In the kitchen there were homemade cookies and candies. The aroma of varnish and wood shavings emanated from my Dad's shop in the basement. There were usually sewing and knitting projects that had to be finished late at night so they would be ready for Christmas.

The days are short in December, and in the midwest, where I grew up, they are often snowy and cold. When school was out, we would tramp the fields and woods around our town and find places to use the toboggan that our parents gave us one Christmas. The cold felt good, especially at the end of the day when we got home to sit by the fire. And the pungent aroma of clove and cinnamon that came drifting from the kitchen was a mouth-watering promise of the cakes, the pies, or the cinnamon rolls that could be found there.

One Christmas I read a story about the Yule Log—the large chunk of timber which in English legend is traditionally set ablaze on Christmas Eve to initiate festivities for the celebration of the holiday. I decided to cut such a log. With an old handsaw we found, I set out to bring home the largest piece of a tree that would fit in the fireplace. I measured the opening with a piece of stick and marked the length by cutting a nick with the edge of my knife. The saw was old and dull; the log was heavy, thick, and damp. It seemed to me that the job of cutting it would take forever. When the cut was finally complete, I hefted my prize and dragged it home. I rolled it into the fireplace and stuffed as much kindling around it as I could cram into the opening. Our Yule Log burned for many hours and brought warmth and cheeriness to the hearth.

Then there was the Christmas tree. In our family we all went together to get the tree. We would pile into the old 1954 Plymouth to go hunting in the Christmas tree lots for just the right one. The various members of the family had different objectives. Dad wanted the tree to be cheap—affordable if you want the polite word. Mom wanted it to be full and pretty. We kids wanted it to be big.

When we arrived at the Christmas tree lot, the kids would spread out in all directions, hunting through the trees. Every few seconds somebody would yell that the perfect specimen had been located. The whole family would come to admire it, and I would be asked to examine it with my hands to see what I thought. The spruce trees were my favorite, the ones with the little short needles and the teeny little pine cones.

When the best of the trees had been discovered, the price negotiations began. This was my father's responsibility. A good tree was one that had plenty of branches, no holes, a height of at least nine feet, no bare spots, and a nice Christmas tree shape. Such a tree was acceptable, but it could be made much better if my father got a "deal." If the asking price for the tree could be reduced by a third or a half, our Christmas tree was one of the best.

We would climb back into the old Plymouth and lean out the windows so Dad could hand us the prized possession. We would drive home slowly, freezing our hands and ears clutching tightly to the tree, which we held pressed to the side of the car. With four or five of us grasping the trunk, the branches of the tree filled the windows on the driver's side of the car. It wasn't easy to see on our side, so we honked the horn a lot at intersections on the way home.

When we arrived home, it was my father's job to set up the tree. Because of a number of disasters (there is a particularly unfortunate Christmas morning that I remember when the tree fell over in the middle of a number of packages) it became the custom in our house to anchor the tree with a cord to at least two separate brackets on the wall.

Then it was time to decorate. This was Mom's special area of interest and talent. She directed all of us in the process and added the finishing touches herself. When the balls were hung, the tinsel meticulously arranged, and the lights lit, the tree changed the living room from a nice place to be to the center of enchantment.

As I remember the Christmases of my growing up years, it is clear to me that my blindness was not a major ingredient. Christmas memories remind me of home and of family members who care for one another. Gentleness, admiration, hope, and faith—of such as these are memorable Christmases made.

I did not know, when I was a student at the school for the blind, what my own life could bring. However, as I prepare for Christmas this year, I am reminded of those joyful experiences of long ago. I now have a family of my own. One of the important ceremonies in our household is the procurement of the Christmas tree.

My son David (a third-grader) asked me to help him build a Christmas present for his Mom. Together we are cutting the wood and fitting the pieces. The staining and finishing must be accomplished before the festive day. The aroma of varnish will mingle this year with the smells of cinnamon and chocolate as we prepare for the giving of gifts.

Perhaps the joy of the season is even greater because there were many times when

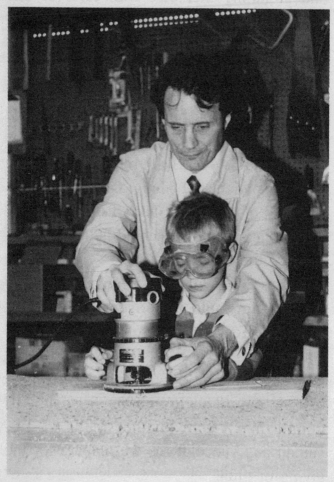

Marc Maurer and his son David work on Christmas present for Mom.

I wondered if it would be available to me. Can blind people have good jobs and raise families? These are questions which come inevitably to the mind of a blind student growing up. They demand answers, but information is scarce, and sometimes the messages are discouraging.

When I came to be a part of the National Federation of the Blind in 1969, I met caring people who were willing to give me the benefit of their knowledge and experience. I met those who had hope and faith. I came to be a part of an organization of individuals who cared for one another.

The responsiveness, the support, the warmth, and the caring I found in the National Federation of the Blind are reminiscent of the gentleness, the faith, and the hope I had come to associate with the Christmas season. I have known the commitment of the National Federation of the Blind for almost a quarter of a century. In that time many thousands of blind people have been given encouragement and support. Many Yule Logs have been cut, and many trees decorated. A number of blind children have come to be blind adults with children of their own. The blindness, which might have prevented a full life, was not permitted to interfere. The Christmases for those blind people have been warm, hearty, hopeful celebrations. We are planning for many more.

BABY-SITTING

by Barbara Walker

In the National Federation of the Blind there are three simple sentences which we have repeated among ourselves and to others so often that they have become more than words and more than slogans. Barbara Walker's story, "Baby-Sitting," is a graphic demonstration of the truth of those three sentences. Read her story. At the end of it you'll find the three sentences I'm talking about. Incidentally, Barbara Walker is one of the finest people I know.

As I hung up the phone, I thought to myself "I bet Sue has no idea what she has just done." To her it was probably just another routine thing to do. But as I told my husband about it, I felt the warmth that true acceptance brings flowing through me and giving a spark to my comments.

"Jim," I said, "Sue just called and suggested that we have our school parent-teacher conferences back to back so I can watch Eric during hers and she can watch Marsha and John during ours. She asked if I would arrange it since she's real busy at work during Larry's free time."

It was a routine call about a routine matter for parents. So what was I so thrilled about? It was the first time anyone had talked to me about watching their children without commenting in some way or expressing some apprehension about my blindness. Sue did tell me later that people had asked her about how she could trust me to watch Eric. She had told them that all she knew was that my children seemed fine and well cared for to her and whenever she wanted to know specifically how I did things she asked.

Unfortunately, Sue is still an exception in this and many other everyday circumstances for the blind. But people like her help people like me deal with the more typical approaches we face, such as that with Chong.

Chong, like Sue and several others, had been providing rides for my children to and from pre-school. Occasionally, she would invite my children to play with hers after school and then bring them home. They enjoyed it, and as they got to know Jenny and Bryan better, wanted to have them to our house. The first couple times I asked Chong about it, the reasons they couldn't seemed plausible. But by the third time, it seemed that perhaps reasons were becoming excuses. My children began wondering aloud why Chong's children couldn't play at our house. At one point, Marsha said she thought Jenny was disappointed about not coming. I thought about blind friends who had talked about this kind of thing. Now it was happening to me. Perhaps we were all paranoid and jumping to conclusions. I thought of Sue and decided we weren't.

The next time I talked to Chong, I said that my children loved to play at her house, but they were wondering why they could never play with Jenny and Bryan at ours. I talked about Jenny's apparent disappointment. Then I took the plunge and asked if my blindness had anything to do with it. She said shyly, "No, not really." I said that if it felt uncomfortable to her, I would be glad to explain how I do things or answer questions. I told her I am used to doing that. She said she didn't have any questions, and we arranged for a time for them to come.

On the day that they were to come, she called and said that Bryan was sleeping late and she would prefer not to wake him. I said we weren't on a schedule that would make their coming later a problem. I was relieved when she agreed to that.

When they arrived, I explained to them in their mother's presence that I was going to put bells on their shirts so I would be able to hear where they were going. I also explained my rule about answering when I call their name unless we were playing hide and seek—something which is only done with everyone knowing before the game starts.

From the time their mother left until she returned, three-year-old Jenny asked almost nonstop questions about my blindness. She wanted to know how I kept track of things, how I got food, how I knew where I was going, how I read stories, how I knew what color things were, how I picked out my clothes, how I washed myself and my children, how I knew who people were, etc. When I changed her two-year-old brother's diaper, she watched with keen interest as I cleaned him and snapped up his clothes. The children all had a good time.

When Chong came to get Jenny and Bryan, I told her what a good time we had all had. I said Jenny had asked a lot of questions and had been very interested in how I do things. I then told her what Jenny had asked and how I had answered. She listened intently, occasionally adding a comment or question of her own. As they prepared to leave, Jenny, who had been in the other room with my daughter during most of Chong's and my conversation, talked excitedly to her mother about my ways of doing things, most of which were just like hers.

I had the distinct impression that Chong and Jenny had wondered to each other about things before coming to our house. Both the bubbly three-year-old and the reserved mother seemed pleased about learning new things, and our relationship thereafter was much more relaxed and comfortable.

Since that time, I have had many opportunities to supervise other people's children. Sometimes the parent or parents have been immediately receptive to trade-offs such as the one Sue initiated with me. Sometimes it has taken direct conversations or recommendations from others to help parents feel comfortable about my watching their children. There continue to be a few who just won't do it.

My perspective on this is that we, through our everyday lives, are making progress. I am glad there are people like Sue to provide a balance for those who won't accept our lives for what they are. Sue and others like her give substance to our acceptance of ourselves as part of the mainstream of society. I also appreciate those like Chong who are willing to listen and change their minds about us. Without them, the progress we're making would not be possible.

Most of all, I applaud children for their willingness to ask questions and remind us that change is occurring through them. As they expect us to take charge, we find it more possible to do so. As they challenge us to live what we say, we reach to do that, too. As we in the National Federation of the Blind share our experiences with each other and with the rest of society, we will find encouragement and the strength to continue to educate ourselves so that the success of acceptance will breed success. It is a privilege to be a part of the process.

As we in the National Federation of the Blind have learned so well, the real problem of blindness is not the loss of eyesight. The real problem is the misunderstanding and lack of information which exist. If a blind person has proper training and opportunity, blindness can be reduced to the level of a physical nuisance.

LET THAT BLIND MAN WORK ON MY TRUCK

by Daryel White

Some of the most lively, interesting, and inspirational agenda items at our national conventions are the presentations made by our own members who are earning their daily bread in occupations that many people would think closed to blind employees. At our recent convention one young man captivated the audience with his story of returning to auto body repair after he became blind. Now meet Daryel White, vice president of the St. Louis County Chapter of the National Federation of the Blind of Missouri and a first-rate employee at Marty's Body Works:

I'm proud to be here today to tell you a little bit about what I do to earn my daily bread. I'll begin by telling you where I was and how I got to where I am today.

I'm from St. Louis, Missouri. Approximately five years ago I lost my eyesight. For about six months I sat and thought I was never going to amount to anything in life. A rehab counselor came to my home, and by the time he left I was even more convinced that I had no future. Then about six months later a rehabilitation teacher knocked on my door. I said, "Who are you?" It had been about six months since the rehab counselor had come, and here she was. She asked me a few questions, which I answered. She said to me, "What did your rehab counselor tell you?"

I said, "Well, he looked at me and said I wasn't going to do anything with my life but be what I call a housewife." At that time I didn't know any different. I had just lost my sight, and I thought maybe that's all I could ever be. This bright young lady really impressed me when she first came into my home. She showed me how to do things that I didn't think I could do, but more than anything else, she told me something I could hardly believe: she said that I could do whatever I wanted to—that I could do what I had done before I became blind.

This lady's name was Patty Page. She introduced me to her brother, a man who has taken me as far as I can go in making my life better. His name is Homer Page, and he is president of the National Federation of the Blind of Colorado and one of the Boulder County Commissioners. I went to meet him while he was visiting at his sister's home. I'll remember this till the day I die; we were sitting at his sister's table, and he asked me what I wanted in life. I told him that I wanted to do what I had been doing when I was sighted—have my own home, have my own job, and live as I was then. He looked at me and said, "You will have that."

I said "o.k." But in my mind I thought, "Well, this guy's really lost it."

He went over to the phone and made a call to a lady who in my heart has really become like my mother.

I first met her in Denver when I came off the plane from St. Louis. I could hardly even walk. I mean I had hold of this stewardess like she was my savior! When I got into the gate area, this woman came up to me and said her name was Diane McGeorge. Then she took me with her—here I am, totally blind, and she says, "I'll take you to get your luggage." And she was totally blind. I thought to myself, "This lady's lost it too!" But I hung on to her because I was frightened. We got the luggage and went to her home, and then I went to the apartments for students at the National Federation of the Blind's Colorado Center for the Blind. Diane McGeorge and Homer Page had managed to enroll me as a student at the Center.

From that moment on I began building my confidence. I learned how to travel. I had had a cane, but I couldn't even find my feet! The staff helped me with cane travel, Braille, and self-confidence. They also introduced me to the organization that is really my support and backbone today—the National Federation of the Blind.

I spent about ten months in Colorado, and toward the end I made some phone calls looking for a job. Even on the day I graduated from the CCB, I made a couple of phone calls and got turned down. But eventually I got lucky with Marty's Body Works, which is in St. Louis, Missouri. I do auto repair, paint cars, and put fenders and doors on. I even do welding.

Now I want to tell you a little story. When I came back from the Colorado Center for the Blind, my confidence level was taller than the highest building that was ever built, so my first job with the public's eye on me was a hard one. I went to work for

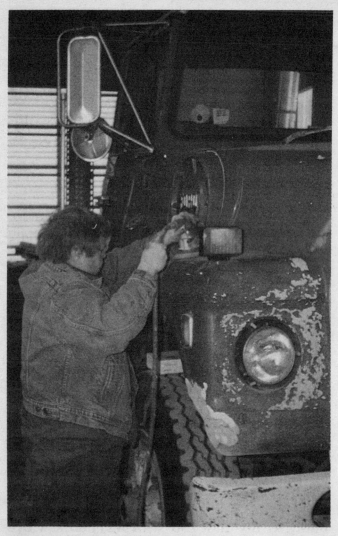

Daryel White on the job.

Marty's Body Works two weeks after I got back from Denver, Colorado.

There's a man named Charlie Collins who owns a big diesel shop in St. Louis. He wrecked his brand new pick-up truck in a front end collision. He had it towed to Marty's. He looked at Marty and he looked at me. Then he said, "I do not, do *not* want that blind man to work on my truck!" Marty looked at me and kind of smiled, and Charlie went on home.

Then Marty said, "Daryel, you're going to do that job." So I brought the truck in and did the job. I put it all together and painted it. I mean, I did a superb job. There was nothing wrong with that truck when I got done.

When Charlie came back to pick it up, Marty told him, "Charlie, I don't want you to pay for that job right now. I know how you are; I've done work for you before. You take the truck back to your shop. I want you to check it over just as close as you can for fender and hood gaps." (These gaps are the distance between the pieces of the car you build or rebuild.) He said, "I want you to bring it back tomorrow and tell me if you find anything wrong."

So Charlie took it to his shop, and he brought it back the next day. He said, "Marty, that's the most fantastic job I've ever seen!"

Marty looked at him, and he looked at me. Then he told Charlie right there, "That is what a blind man can do."

Charlie owns two eighteen-wheelers over the road. About two weeks later he wrecked one of his eighteen-wheelers. He brought it back to Marty's, and do you know what his first words were? "Let that blind man work on my truck."

I want everyone to know one thing: I thank you for the support of the NFB, of all you people who are listening to me and holding this organization together. People like Dr. Jernigan, President Maurer, Diane

McGeorge, and Homer Page are the ones that really have made me the person I am today.

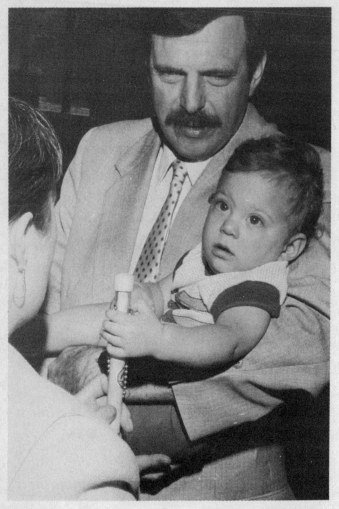

Stephen Benson with his son, Patrick.

BLUEPRINT FOR LEARNING?

by Stephen O. Benson

In many ways a great deal of progress has been made by blind people in recent times—more jobs, better special tools and equipment, increased understanding. But in at least one critical area blind children growing up today are being very badly short-changed in a way that was very nearly unheard of when I was a child in the mid-1930s. In recent decades most blind children have not routinely been taught how to read and write Braille. Many of these children have now reached adulthood. I talk to them by the hundreds. Almost without exception they feel they were betrayed by their teachers and the other "experts" their parents trusted to plan their education.

We as blind people should not have to fight for blind children to have the chance to learn to read and write Braille.

Parents expect schools to teach sighted children how to read and write, and there are laws requiring that it be done. We want the laws to protect blind children, too. But the "experts" often fight against such laws. They seem to think deciding whether to teach a blind child to read Braille is very complicated. The truth is that it is very simple. If a child can't see well enough to read print easily, Braille should be taught. But that is not what usually happens, and the blind child pays a heavy price for the rest of his or her life.

Stephen Benson is totally blind and is President of the National Federation of the Blind of Illinois. In "Blueprint for Learning," he describes in vivid detail the "experts'" decisions which crippled his early education. Unfortunately his experience is still being repeated in countless lives across our country.

At one and a half years of age my eye condition was diagnosed as retinitis pigmentosa, which often results in total blindness. As I approached first grade, my doctors and teachers (the team of professionals) asserted that I should use my limited vision to its maximum for as long as possible. My family was directed to enroll me in what was then called "sight saving." Print was to be the medium by which I was to learn to read.

The sight saving classroom was equipped with the best technology of the day (1948): dark green chalkboards with yellow chalk, yellow paper with heavy green lines, indirect lighting, desks with adjustable work surfaces that allowed the student to bring reading and writing materials closer to the face, and typewriters with large print. Each student wore prescription lenses and had access to hand-held magnifiers. In addition we used large-print textbooks. In third grade we learned to type by the touch typing method.

In my case and in countless others, neither equipment nor teaching techniques would or could work. The techniques and the teachers' efforts were misapplied. The prescription for sight saving class was in error. From the first day of class my limited vision prevented me from reading effectively. Over the course of the next four and a half years my visual acuity decreased while the print I was expected to read became smaller.

I remember alternately gazing out the window and puzzling over a printed page. By fourth grade my teachers had to print out my class work by hand, using large letters and india ink. With all of that I still felt as though I was reading grey print on grey paper. Yet I remained in sight saving class until the middle of fifth grade.

The toll I paid for the professionals' decisions was high. I dreaded reading; my confidence eroded; I feared blindness; I acquired bad reading habits that carried over into adulthood. I never checked a book out of the library. Why should I? I couldn't read it.

During the summer of 1952 the professionals finally admitted that print might not be the right way for me to be getting an education. In September of that year I was transferred to what we referred to as the blind school, where I began to learn Braille. It wasn't difficult. My teacher was competent. She knew Braille. She gave me positive encouragement. My reading and writing speeds were slow at first; however, as I gained proficiency and confidence, speeds increased. In January of 1953, at age eleven, I checked out and read a library book for the first time in my life. It was in Braille.

Over the last forty years teams of professionals have continued to make the same foolish and costly decisions, probably with greater frequency as the years have passed.

As a member of the National Federation of the Blind's Scholarship Committee, I have met an astounding number of high school and college students who, because they had <u>some</u> vision, were deprived of Braille or were discouraged from learning it without regard to whether the student could read print well enough to compete with sighted peers.

One scholarship applicant, not unusual, uses taped books and a closed circuit television magnifier. Under the best conditions she is able to read for only a minute at a time, and that with great discomfort. She is enrolled as a part-time student in a community college, partly because her vision doesn't allow her to meet the reading and writing demands of full-time status. She has asked to be taught Braille, but her family and the teams of professionals with whom she has worked have actively discouraged it.

Too many parents assume that the "experts" must "know what's best," and will necessarily "do what's best for the child." Those assumptions are often wrong and prove to be quite costly to the blind child.

"What's best for the child" is a catch phrase that too often translates into decisions that are convenient for the teacher, school, or district and into efforts to make the blind child's educational needs conform to budget priorities.

Were my experience forty years ago and that of the college student I described mere coincidence? I don't believe they were. Nor do I believe that de-emphasis on literacy (Braille) was or is accidental.

De-emphasis on Braille is disgraceful, just as de-emphasis on print would be. People who have a good command of reading and writing skills tend to do better in math, science, history, languages, music, and all the rest. People who can read and write successfully have a better chance at competitive employment and every other situation in life, for that matter.

The anti-literacy/anti-Braille position taken by so many educators of blind children and adults has had wider negative impact than they might imagine. Several years ago, I worked at an agency for the blind in Chicago. In support of a program to teach Braille, I submitted a grant request to the Chicago Tribune Foundation. The grant request was turned down. The reasons, according to a foundation spokesman, were that Braille has nothing to do with literacy, it is obsolete, and reading can be done by recordings.

I was disappointed that the program did not receive that support. I was disgusted by the ignorance of the foundation personnel, but I was not surprised.

For fifteen years I taught Braille for the Veterans Administration at Hines Hospital. One of my assigned duties was to supervise Western Michigan University interns (student teachers), studying to become rehabilitation teachers.

An alarming number of these interns didn't know Grade II Braille, could not write with a slate and stylus, and had to be instructed in the use of an ordinary Braille writer. One intern didn't know Grade I Braille, though he had taken and passed a Braille course.

Though I wrote negative reports regarding their poor skills, all of these interns passed the internship, and presumably all were certified by the Association for the Education and Rehabilitation of the Blind and Visually Impaired (AER).

If future generations of blind people, children and adults, are to be literate, if future generations of blind people hope to be competitive in society, they _must_ have access to the printed word by a method that will allow _writing_ as well as reading. It is time for educators to grit their teeth and admit that a colossal error has been made.

Then they must bring themselves up to speed on Braille and all of its tools, mechanical and electronic. It is time for educators to join us in our effort to require that Braille be made available to any child who wants it and to participate in making sure that sufficient funding is available to make mandates and good intentions mean something.

SUCCESSFUL EQUATION: SKILLS + CONFIDENCE = SUCCESS

by Tom Ley

Tom Ley was a 1987 National Federation of the Blind scholarship winner. Here is what he has to say about his progression from frightened high school senior rapidly becoming blind to confident high school math teacher:

I grew up as a sighted kid and always wanted to be a football player. At least, I wanted this career until I was ten or so. Due to diabetes, I started to become blind during my last year of high school. It took about ten months to go from having twenty-twenty vision to being totally blind. During that year I went through many of the experiences other people have who are losing their sight. My grades started going down, and I made a trip to the college I had chosen in order to learn my way around the campus while I still had some sight. At that time I did not know about the National Federation of the Blind. Therefore, I did a lot of suffering: I was falling down stairs, and I could not read room numbers. I did not know that blind persons have alternative ways of solving such problems.

I had wanted to be an electrical engineer. When I went blind, my father looked in a reference book, where he found a list of jobs the book's author presumed a blind person could do. Among the jobs was electrical engineering. I had been blind for only a few months, and I did not know any blind people. I thought I was very lucky that I could continue in my chosen career.

After high school I got some training in the skills of blindness. In Arkansas I was taught how to use a very short cane and learned to read Braille, and then I came back to Louisiana and enrolled in college.

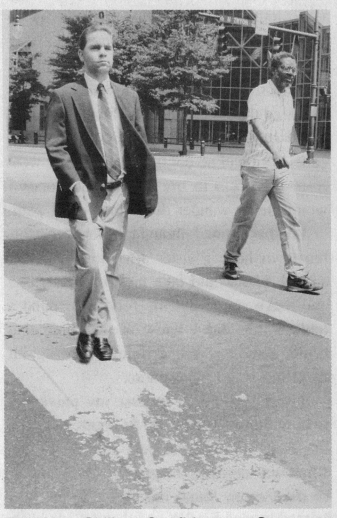

Tom Ley: Skills + Confidence = Success.

I really enjoyed my course work at Louisiana Tech, and I was doing rather well. But I did not have enough of the skills of blindness, so I was having to study twice as much as the other students. For that reason I had no social life. I knew how to use a cane, but I had no confidence. I simply went from my dorm to my classes and hoped I would never wander down the wrong path.

At that point I thought I was very fortunate to have a sister attending the same school. She would take me to the cafeteria and make sure I got my food and found a table. Little did I know at that time that blind persons were efficiently doing all these tasks and many more.

I was very lucky because my university is in the town of Ruston. At about that time the Federation's Louisiana Center for the Blind was opening. Joanne Wilson, Director of the Center, found me and took me to a state convention of the National Federation of the Blind of Louisiana.

At that convention I saw a lot of normal blind people. If you took away their blindness and the alternative techniques they used, you would consider them just average folks. These blind people were doing things that normal people do. When I was with them, I knew that they had something I wanted. At that point I decided that I needed the special training which I had not been offered previously.

At about that same time I began realizing that maybe engineering was not what I really wanted to do. I was looking at the engineering jobs my classmates were getting, and I noticed that they lacked the human interaction I wanted. I had always enjoyed teaching, doing tutoring when I was in high school. The idea struck me that I would like to be a teacher. But I had never heard of a high school math teacher who was blind. I thought it was out of the question.

I wanted to be just like the high school math teachers I had had, and I did not want to teach at a school for the blind. There is nothing wrong with teaching at a blind school, but I wanted to be right in the mainstream. At first I did not think I could really do the job. I figured that I could do some of the tasks, but not all, and I did not think anyone would hire me.

I started at the Louisiana Center for the Blind in 1988. I had attended my first National Convention in 1987, where I was a scholarship winner. I attended my first National Association of Blind Educators meeting that year. I went around and talked to blind educators. They were employed, so they told me how they accomplished their tasks. They gave me the confidence to believe that, if they could teach, I could too.

At the Louisiana Center I acquired personal confidence, undoubtedly the most important characteristic of all. Until that time I had never had it. I had seen it in other blind people, and I knew that it might be mine, maybe in the future. But because I acquired confidence at that Center, I knew that I could teach. I learned that my blindness is just another part of me as is my height or my being right-handed. Blindness is no longer something which overwhelms me or predominates in my life. It is not the defining factor in my personality.

I enrolled in the department of education at Louisiana Tech. There were no open complaints to my entering; however, the professors let it be known in subtle ways that they had doubts about my ability. I paid no attention to them. I worked my way through the courses and did just fine. Because I did not question my ability to become a math teacher, my confidence was projected to all my professors.

As time went on, my professors decided that blindness was no big deal, for I was doing everything all the other students were doing.

When my master teacher for student teaching learned that a blind student was assigned to him, he was convinced that it would not work. But I showed him that he was wrong. I completed my student teaching and was looking for a job. I was very happy when I got my resumes just like all the other job seekers. But I can tell you all that I would not have gotten anywhere without my confidence, which came from the NFB and the members of the National Association of Blind Educators.

My first year of teaching was challenging, exciting, interesting, and fun. There were a lot of sleepless nights and hard work. Grades and papers must be turned in on time. If grades are due today, no teacher can expect to get extra time. The skills I use in the classroom are basic. My equipment consists of a slate and stylus, a tape recorder, and masking tape. I put the tape on the boards for writing in straight lines. When it came to putting up a graph, I made a grid using my tape and my cane to insure I made the lines straight. I have a computer at home for keeping grades and making tests.

I have the duties of a full-time teacher, including chaperoning the prom. I work selling popcorn at the basketball games and fix the broken popcorn machine too. I am comfortable doing all this, and I know that this is all part of teaching. I received all the skills that helped me get my job from the National Federation of the Blind. I'm excited to be in this organization.

Recently I had a chance to talk to a physics teacher, who has been teaching a long time, but who will be starting his first year as a blind teacher next fall. We all help each other. Together we can demonstrate that, given training and opportunity, blind people can compete successfully in all areas of education.

I REMEMBER

by Mary Ellen Halverson

Mrs. Halverson graduated from the University of Iowa with a major in Spanish. She has taught Spanish in the elementary schools and is now a Braille teacher and an active volunteer in the National Federation of the Blind. She and her husband, Raymond, have two children. Her story, "I Remember," sounds a familiar theme to readers of earlier Kernel Books. How different life would be for the blind child growing up, if parents and teachers had accurate information about blindness. Here is her story:

When I look back on my high school years and consider all of the negative ideas I absorbed about blindness, I really wonder how I survived with any self-respect left at all. I'm sure one reason I did is that I had a very positive, supportive family who believed in me and expected me to do well in school and other activities. Fortunately, in my first year of college I met several young active blind students who began the process of teaching me a whole new attitude about blindness.

I began losing my sight in junior high due to a disease in the retina. When I had long reading assignments, my parents would read them to me in the evening. Many times I had difficulty in reading the blackboard or tests, but I struggled along. I can remember worrying about tests—not about the subject matter to be tested, but about the quality of the mimeographed pages of the test. I knew that frequently the print was faded or blurry and I was reluctant to use a magnifying glass in front of my fellow junior high students.

Some teachers were very helpful, but others seemed not to notice or not be especially concerned. I preferred as little discussion on the matter as possible. Neither my parents nor I realized that by eighth or ninth grade I was definitely legally blind. We told ourselves and others that I just had a "sight problem."

By the time I entered high school, I had lost a little more sight and was enrolled in the Sight Saving program in our school district. My parents and I were quite relieved since this program provided books on tape for me, and a lot of material in large print. There were different types of magnifiers available, and such things as large print dictionaries. However, the only skill I was actually taught by one of the sight saving teachers was typing; which is a valuable skill to have.

I attended my regular high school classes in the morning and then went to a resource room for the afternoon. At first, this room was in an elementary school, which I found rather embarrassing. I traveled there every day with several other students by cab.

Eventually the resource room was moved into the high school which was an improvement.

I remember the first day I met the sight saving teacher, who was a very kind, well-meaning person. Right away she told my family and me that "we never use the word 'blind', we say, 'partially sighted'." This suited us quite well since the word "blind" conjured up terrible and frightening visions in our minds. She further reassured us that I would not have to learn Braille, but could use large print books.

I should tell you right here that in order for me to read even the large print, I had to put my face right down on the page and even then, I could only read several letters at a time. I can remember spending three hours trying to read a chemistry chapter in a large print book one evening. I imagine my fellow students read and studied the chapter in thirty minutes. Although we didn't realize it at the time, Braille would have been much more efficient and faster for me to use. Braille is not an inferior reading system, and can be easily learned.

Another area which caused me some anguish was traveling about both in the school building and outside. It was especially hard to see the down stairs, and I could not read the room numbers. When I approached the stairs I just slowed down and probably looked rather awkward.

I developed my own techniques for finding the right room, such as the second room past the drinking fountain or the room next to the main front door. I did not attend many school or social activities at night because I could not see after dark. My excuse to people was usually that I had to study. Therefore, I missed out on dances, dates, and sports events; all of which are an important part of high school life.

Now I know that this area of travel could have been solved so easily with some training in the use of the long white cane. However, this would not have been successful without some changes in my attitude first. It would have been essential for me to believe that it was respectable to use a white cane. I'm absolutely sure that the resource teachers would have frowned on such ideas. They felt it was best to use one's remaining eyesight as much as possible, even though it was often far less efficient and more painful than alternatives such as Braille and cane travel.

I am now convinced that the key to being an independent, successful, and happy blind person is your attitude about yourself. Along with attitude, but secondary, you must also learn some skills like typing, Braille, cane travel and other techniques that will work for you. During my high school years I had neither the positive attitude about myself nor the skills. I suppose the sad part is that there was no one to teach them to me.

My classroom teachers were sympathetic for the most part, but they could offer no real encouragement or worthwhile advice concerning blindness. In some of my classes I felt that I was a nuisance to the teacher. I was very apologetic when I had to ask to have something read from the blackboard or from a test. You can imagine what this did for my self-esteem!

It was also embarrassing to me to read and write in the classroom because I had to get so close to the paper. A student in one class made a remark I have always remembered. I was writing answers to a quiz and he said, "Now, that's the direct approach." Another blow to one's self-respect. Until this writing, I have never told anyone about that painful moment.

By now I'm sure you can understand how all of these experiences can cause a young person to feel very inferior to her peers. Even though my grades were high my self-respect was low. Of course, I did not realize this at the time.

I should add here that my high school experience was not totally gloomy. I did have a good group of friends, some very cooperative teachers, and a terrific family. I graduated high in my class of 528 classmates and went on to the University. I entered college prepared to struggle on as before, but the unexpected happened.

I met several well-adjusted, confident blind students who had received training in the skills of blindness and had acquired that all-important attitude I mentioned earlier. They knew without a doubt that they were equal to anyone and they were willing to take on their share of responsibilities both in school and any other area of life.

They also had another thing in common—they were members of the National Federation of the Blind and met for monthly meetings. At first I tried to avoid these meetings since I did not wish to admit that I was blind. But on the other hand, I liked these friends personally, and I wanted the same confidence and freedom they possessed.

After a couple of years of college I attended an orientation and adjustment center which taught skills and began the long process of improving my attitude toward myself and my blindness. It was, beyond a doubt, the most valuable year of my life. Very few places and very few people can restore a person's self-dignity and respect so effectively.

Sometimes I think about how those teenage years might have been. I also think about the young people who are living my experiences right now, and about their parents who are worried and don't know what to do. If my story reaches you and helps any of you in one small way, those years of worry and embarrassment will have all been worth it!

Parents, your children who are partially or totally blind, do have the opportunity to become independent, happy and successful individuals. It is respectable to be blind.

BLINDNESS AND THE BROOKLYN BRIDGE

By Kenneth Silberman

What does blindness have to do with the Brooklyn Bridge? Let Kenneth Silberman tell you:

I grew up in Cheltenham, Pennsylvania, a suburb of Philadelphia. At the age of five, I entered kindergarten just like all the other kids, but something was different. I couldn't see as much detail or see as far as the others. No matter, I was still participating in all the activities of the class without serious difficulty.

Grades one through six were a different ball game altogether. Reading, writing, and arithmetic are subjects that require the use of written symbols. For the sighted, this means print, written on sheets of paper, in books, or on the blackboard. In order to read print at all, I needed large print, magnification, or had to sit up close to the board. No matter which technique I employed, I couldn't read very fast or for very long. As the years rolled by, the workload increased, and I had more and more trouble keeping up. It was true that I couldn't see very well, but I was sighted (at least that was what I thought) and should have been able to keep up. But I couldn't and felt stupid because of that fact. I developed an increasing sense of inferiority with each passing year.

In September of my ninth-grade year, I lost my remaining sight. At the time, I thought a catastrophe had befallen me. (I did not yet know about the National Federation of the Blind.) I was blind, but I wasn't going to admit it. I used a cane as little as I could and never indoors.

After all, the last thing I wanted to do was to walk around with a badge of blindness in my hand. Braille was a badge too, and I wasn't going to have anything to do with it either. Besides, it was slow. And after all, there were tape recorders for reading and taking notes. Never mind that I could not keep up and that I could not follow the math, spell, or punctuate. I was blind, and I was doing the best that I could. These were my thoughts at the time. With a few delays, I continued puttering along in this way through my undergraduate years and most of my graduate years as well.

I was really depressed by this time because I couldn't perform assignments in a timely manner, travel by myself, or do much of anything independently. Blindness was a pretty raw deal, or so I thought.

As I now know but didn't then, the characteristic of blindness wasn't the real problem. Rather, my attitudes about blindness were the real raw deal. I remember walking down the hall one day in high school, and a passing teacher remarked, "I can't tell you're blind." I thought this was a real compliment at the time. As I look back on those early years, I realize that I did not think of myself as blind nor did I understand what it means to be blind.

As a result of this mistaken notion, I denied myself the tools that would have helped me to succeed. If I had accepted and understood my blindness, I would have decided to use Braille as my primary reading and writing medium, since a good Braille reader can read three hundred to four hundred words per minute, and would have appreciated print as a helpful aid. I also would have used a white cane since it would have kept me from tripping over and walking into things.

I discovered after a number of painful lessons that it's better to find things with a cane than with your face. By using these techniques, I would have been able to keep right in step with the crowd. Later, when I lost the remainder of my sight, I would have been able to keep right on going without missing a beat. But of course, I knew none of this, and I could not have been expected to.

I was at my lowest emotional point in 1985 when I applied for and won a scholarship from the National Federation of the Blind. I needed money, so I applied. When I arrived at the national convention in Louisville, Kentucky, I found, much to my astonishment, blind people who were happy and successful.

They were traveling about with facility and were reading and writing Braille as deftly as sighted people use print, and they were using these skills to hold down responsible jobs, run households, etc. It was at this time that I started to understand that blindness was not my problem; my attitudes about blindness were the problem.

I had thought the skills of blindness were inferior because they didn't appear on the surface to be like those of the sighted. Hence, I had thought the blind were inferior; I had thought I was inferior. And so, I had denied my blindness. (You must understand. I had only known sighted people up to this point.) But the evidence was clear. The alternative techniques of blindness enable us to live full and rich lives just as the sighted do. I now realize that while the money was very helpful, I received a much more valuable gift, The National Federation of the Blind.

I had a choice. I could either deal with the situation or continue as before. I decided to get to work. I picked up some books on Braille and set about learning it. It was hard to go to school and learn Braille at the same time, but I knew that I had to either learn it or drop out. The latter was not acceptable, and I couldn't deal with things as they were any longer.

By the time I graduated, I was doing much of my school work in Braille. I continued to use taped books and readers in conjunction with Braille. All these techniques have their place. In January, 1987, I received my Master's Degree in Aerospace Engineering from Cornell University.

After graduation, I enrolled in a rehabilitation program in order to develop my Braille and cane skills. I continued to work on my outlook toward blindness by drawing strength from my new-found Federation friends.

Finally, it was time to look for a job. After a little more than a year, I secured employment with the U.S. Navy in Philadelphia. I really got the opportunity to test my newly-developed skills and my mettle in that job. I had had only one computer course in college and was now expected to learn how to write databases on the job. I did it. This is quite an accomplishment for anyone, blind or sighted.

Today, I work as an administrator/engineer for the National Aeronautics and Space administration. I manage the Publications group for the National Space Science Data Center. This means that I am respon-

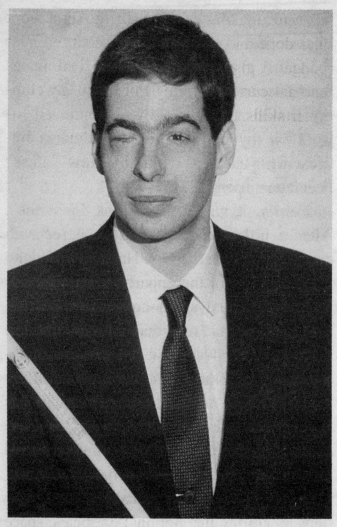

Kenneth Silberman

sible for making sure that the group's work gets done and that the work comes in under budget. I also serve on various committees and am currently trying to expand my computer skills.

How do my alternative techniques compare with those of my sighted colleagues? Let's compare a few of them. I use a reader to help me with paperwork; my boss uses a secretary. My co-workers take notes with pens and pencils; I use a slate and stylus to write Braille. My colleagues use a computer with the help of a monitor and a printer; I use a computer with the help of a speech synthesizer and a Braille embosser. My fellow employees travel about safely with the help of sight; I travel about safely with the help of my white cane. The sighted have techniques that work for them, and the blind have techniques that work equally well.

My professional objective is to become a senior administrator in America's space program. In reaching that goal, I will be helping to build upon the foundation, the record of achievement and success, built by past generations of Federationists. Those who came before us worked to give us the opportunities that we have today. It is up to us to make life better for future generations of blind people.

I still don't have all of the skills and self-confidence that I need, but I am working on it. I am able to improve myself because I now see blindness for what it is, a characteristic, a mere physical nuisance. By utilizing the alternative techniques of blindness, I can and do compete on equal terms with my sighted colleagues.

When the Brooklyn Bridge was built [1869-1883], engineers of the day said that it couldn't be done. John Augustus Roebling and his son, Colonel Washington Roebling, believed that it could, and they had the know-how to build it. The real obstacle to the project was not the techniques needed to build the Bridge. Rather, it was the entrenched, traditional ideas of the engineering community. But the Roeblings knew the truth. They had the knowledge and the leadership to go beyond the conventional wisdom of their day. Were they right? The answer spans the East River today, more than a century after its construction.

We, the blind of the nation, have the know-how to lead full and rich lives. Like the Roeblings, we have to believe in ourselves and need to have the leadership to make our dreams of equality come true. Since 1940, we have encouraged and supported each other. Since 1940, we have shared our collective know-how. And since 1940, we have had the leadership to climb within reach of equality and first-class citizenship. In other words, since 1940, we have had the National Federation of the Blind.

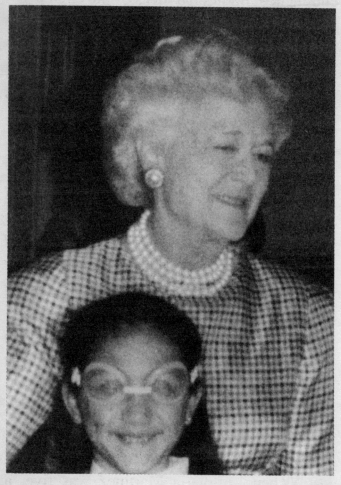

Lisamaria in 1990 with First Lady Barbara Bush.

LISAMARIA: FOCUSING ON OTHERS

In the August 11, 1992, issue of Woman's Day, an article appeared which profiled the lives of several children with disabilities who have not let their problems stand in their way. Barbara Bartocci, the author of the article, contacted us to ask if we could suggest the name of a blind child for this profile. Without hesitation we suggested Lisamaria Martinez and her family. Lisamaria's mother is one of the leaders of the California Parents of Blind Children Division of the National Federation of the Blind. And NFB philosophy has been a part of the Martinez family's thoughts and actions for several years. The results are unmistakable. Now meet Lisamaria Martinez:

When Lisamaria Martinez was five, a strange rash, followed by blisters, erupted all over her body. Her temperature soared to 105 degrees, and her eyes swelled shut. "She could die," the doctor warned her terrified parents, as they rushed the pretty girl to the hospital.

In the next few weeks Lisamaria's blisters broke open, and her skin slithered off. Clumps of her waist-length hair fell out. She couldn't bear to open her eyes to light or air; it hurt too much.

As Lisamaria's world grew dark, doctors diagnosed her mysterious ailment, a rare skin condition called Stevens-Johnson syndrome. Greg and Maria Martinez learned the worst: their daughter was permanently blind. Just twenty-eight and twenty-seven years old, the young couple lived in Oceanside, California, a continent away from their families in Puerto Rico. Lisamaria was the older of their two daughters. They were devastated.

Yet Maria Martinez also felt profound gratitude. She had told her husband, during the awful days when they feared Lisamaria might die, "God gave our daughter to us, and God can take her back; it's not for us to say." God had returned their daughter; surely they could deal with blindness.

Since her eyes no longer could tear, Lisamaria had to wear protective goggles day and night. "In first grade everyone stared at me," she relates matter-of-factly. "Sometimes they were mean—we had crayon holders at our desks, and I couldn't tell which color was which, so I'd ask for help, and kids gave me the wrong color on purpose."

As Lisamaria learned to navigate with her cane, Greg encouraged her to go wherever she wanted to go. The Martinezes treated Lisamaria as normally as they did her younger sister.

In second grade Lisamaria entered the annual National Federation of the Blind's "Braille Readers Are Leaders" contest. "I'm going to win!" she boasted to her parents, and they encouraged her determination. In three months, she read sixty-two books, winning her division.

By third grade Lisamaria joined Brownies and, pushing her cane ahead of her, hiked up trails with her friends. She also found an outlet for what her father calls a "natural desire to help people." In Brownies she collected canned goods for homeless shelters and visited the elderly in hospitals. At school she volunteered to pick up trash. "I got my friends to help," she admits.

The efforts of a nine-year-old blind girl to help the elderly caught public attention. In 1990 Lisamaria was nominated for the national Kiwanis Hope of America Award and, later that year, was named California's recipient of the coveted Jefferson Awards for Students for her community service. Lisamaria and her mother flew to Washington, D.C., for the presentation, and there, says Lisamaria proudly, "I got my picture taken with Mrs. Bush." It doesn't bother her that she can't see the photo.

Lisamaria still has trying times—in physical education, for instance. "It's hard to bat and run bases when you're blind, but my teacher says she'll blindfold everyone in my class someday so they'll understand what it's like."

Most important: Lisamaria doesn't feel sorry for herself. "Nothing holds her back" says her mother. "When I see her running on the playground, she is just like a normal child. Her attitude is: 'It might take me longer, but I can do whatever I want to do.'"

ON THE STIGMA OF BLINDNESS

by Michael Freeman

Michael Freeman and his wife Barbara live in the state of Washington, where Michael is a computer programmer for a large utility company. Here he writes thoughtfully of a small incident, which deepened his and his wife's understanding of the ingrained public attitudes about blindness.

Throughout history blindness has been misunderstood by almost everyone. The word "blind" has had connotations of helplessness, witlessness and lack of discernment. Blindness has been (and still is, to some extent) considered a stigma and a badge of shame; for this reason many blind persons are hesitant to admit that they are blind and try to avoid any action such as reading Braille or carrying a cane which would categorize them as blind.

Every thoughtful blind person is aware of this stigma. Indeed, although I acknowledged its existence, I rejected it from an early age. Joining the National Federation of the Blind only increased my awareness of this stigma and strengthened my resolve to overcome it. However, its impact was brought home to my wife and me when we were on a trip a number of years ago. We had gone to the National Center for the Blind, headquarters of the National Federation of the Blind, in Baltimore, Maryland, to participate in a leadership seminar. We flew on United Airlines, making a change of planes in Chicago. I had traveled to the seminar using an aluminum cane; while in Baltimore, I bought an NFB fiberglass cane. On the return trip, therefore, I carried two canes.

We again had to change planes in Chicago. My wife, who is sighted, offered to carry one of my canes as I had my hands full with a briefcase and the other cane. Neither of us was prepared for her reaction. As we walked together between concourses, she felt strange and extremely conspicuous. It was late at night and we were the only people walking the corridors. It made no difference. She felt self-conscious and uncomfortable.

My wife considered herself a staunch Federationist and, intellectually, at least, had embraced the concept that it is respectable to be blind. Nevertheless, when put to the test, the indoctrination of a lifetime came to the fore and she felt, if not shame, at least discomfort that she might be viewed as blind.

The story does not end here, however. As the years have passed, my wife has carried canes for me on several occasions with little thought or notice. Since she has now met hundreds of competent blind people, the experience of carrying a cane no longer produces a painful negative reaction; my wife has come to view blindness as a characteristic—one of many exhibited by humankind and of which a person need not be ashamed. Indeed, we have experienced in our own lives the truth of the Federation statement that it is respectable to be blind and that we in the National Federation of the Blind are changing what it means to be blind.

CLIMB EVERY MOUNTAIN

by Barbara Pierce

How does a blind person overcome a lifetime of conditioning that tells you that if you are blind, you can't. Can't what? Can't whatever it is, no matter what. One way is by choosing some unusual activity (like mountain climbing, for example) that everyone <u>knows</u> a blind person can't do— and then doing it. At the National Federation of the Blind's training center in Colorado, this is exactly what we do. Here is how Barbara Pierce, who is totally blind, describes the experience:

Everyone talks about the beauty of the Rockies, but somehow I was unprepared for it when I, along with several other blind people, arrived at the International Alpine School to go rock climbing. We were fitted with climbing boots, harnesses, and hard hats. Stowing this equipment, our water bottles, and lunches in our backpacks, we began hiking.

The air was incredibly clear, and though it was hot, the shade was cool and the breeze invigorating. There were thousands of birds who had had the good sense to take up residence in this ruggedly beautiful country, and not many insects. Much of the way we were accompanied by a noisy little stream rushing over rocks and generally adding a great deal to our appreciation of the place.

The guides had been busy before our arrival placing ropes at several points on rock faces for us to climb. As far as I could gather, this entailed someone's climbing without the protection of a rope to the top of the rock to fix an anchor into the ground, through which the rope was then passed.

When one of us decided to try a particular climb, an experienced climber would sit down at the bottom and control one end of the rope. The other end was passed through the special loops on the novice climber's harness and tied securely and quite mysteriously. We were shown how to tie these knots, but I, for one, was happy to let the experts do the job for me. Then, with the rope securely connecting climber to stationary belayer by way of the anchor at the top of the rock, one began to climb.

The early rock faces had obvious hand and foot holds as well as some slant. These were steeper scrambles than I had ever tried before, but with a rope and climbing boots, they were physically taxing but not hard.

Then came an all but vertical rock face with a few—a very few—cracks in it. The people from the climbing school protested that these were not very challenging, but they seemed pretty formidable to us. The picture shown here is of me walking backwards down this climb—a process which requires the climber to lean backwards until he or she is perpendicular to the rock face.

The rope holds the climber in this position, enabling him or her to walk backwards down the distance that has so laboriously been crawled up. My grin in this picture is a measure of the exhilaration I felt after having pitted myself against the rock and won.

Those of us who wanted to try something even more difficult were then directed to a small cliff—I use the word advisedly. It was absolutely vertical, and there was almost nothing to stand on.

I did not get more than ten or twelve feet off the ground, though at the time that seemed quite an accomplishment. My undoing came while I was sprawled across the rock. My left foot was more or less anchored in a shallow hollow in the rock, and my hands were spread wide far above my head, clinging to outcrops that were no wider than a quarter of an inch.

The guide who was holding my rope said in a calm (not to say placid) voice, "Now find a place to put your right foot," (which was, as I remember it, flailing around in a frantic effort to do just that). She told me to look higher, that there was a nice hold about two feet above my out-thrust foot.

Eventually, I found what she was talking about. It is no exaggeration to say that the crack in question was at the level of my right shoulder. When I got my foot up there, it felt like it was above my head. Then the guide said, "Now, just transfer your weight to your right foot."

She was so calm about it, as if such a thing could be done. I suggested that she had better begin singing "Climb Every Mountain," and several folks obligingly began doing so. This was the point at which the absurdity of the situation made me begin to laugh, and I peeled off the rock and hung there, helpless with laughter.

My guide told me to rest before trying again. I did so, but by this time my limbs were shaking with fatigue, and eventually I asked her to lower me to the ground.

If I had been a member of a real class, however, I would not have been able to get off so easily. For the only time that day I was glad that I was not engaged in a real rock-climbing course.

This entire experience is a small jewel in my personal collection of memories. Beauty; the camaraderie of adventure shared with good friends; the encouragement and help of warm, calm, and unsentimental experts; and the exhilaration of testing myself against a formidable challenge: these things set that day apart in my memory.

I can readily understand how valuable a whole course of rock-climbing would be as a part of a rehabilitation program. One emerges from such an experience more confident and self-assured. This is the very essence of rehabilitation.

One word must be said about the International Alpine School and its staff who are dedicated to providing climbing experience to blind people. They and their other instructors are wonderful people to work with. They begin with the premise that all climbers can benefit from experience on the rocks. They are unflappable and very encouraging, but above all, they are inspiring climbers, who believe that there is no reason why blind people can't learn to climb well too.

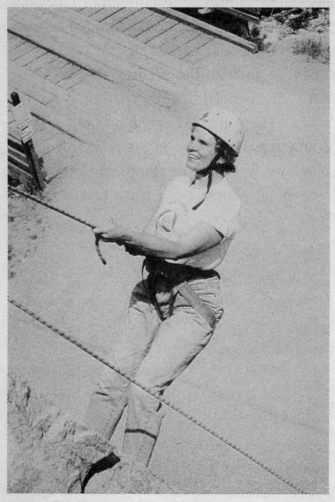

Barbara Pierce works her way up the mountain.

National Federation of the Blind
YOU CAN HELP US...

- Publicize our nationwide annual contest (similar to a summer reading program for sighted children through a local public library) which encourages blind children to compete against one another in the reading of pages of Braille books.

- Publicize our scholarship program for deserving blind students.

- Make books about the capabilities of blind persons available to local public libraries of schools and universities, and distribute films and other literature about positive attitudes about blindness for school and other gatherings.

- Recruit volunteers interested in reading or driving for blind persons, or assisting with shopping needs.

- Conduct or attend Job Opportunities for the Blind (JOB) seminars for prospective blind employees and job applicants to teach the skills of resume writing, job hunting, interviewing, and choosing the appropriate field of work.

- Plan seminars for prospective employers of blind persons to broaden employers' awareness of the capabilities of blind persons and to help eliminate artificial barriers and unfounded prejudice about employing the blind.

WE CARE ABOUT YOU TOO!

- If a family member, friend, or someone you know needs assistance with problems of blindness, please write:

Marc Maurer, President
1800 Johnson Street, Suite 300,
Baltimore, MD 21230-4998
Your contribution is tax-deductible.